RAJA YOGA

YOGA AS MEDITATION!

BESTSELLING AUTHOR

Shreyananda Natha

Cover & Graphic Design

Mattias Långström

Contact: oneofakindbooks@bhagwan.se

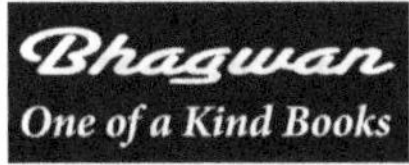

RAJA YOGA

YOGA AS MEDITATION!

BESTSELLING AUTHOR

Shreyananda Natha

ISBN: 9789180207324

✳ ✳ ✳

Publisher: *BHAGWAN 2021*

NAMASTÉ

I want to thank the teachers and students I have had over the years and who have made my journey with yoga so interesting. Thank you for all the inspiration you have given me and for making this book possible. The yoga masters who no longer live among us, live on with every new person who immerses themselves in the yoga tradition.

Sri Swami Sivananda, Sri Swami Satyananda, Sri Tirumalai Krishnamacharya, Sri Swami Vishnudevananda, Sri K. Pattabhi Jois, Osho, Swami Nirdosha, Swami Omananda, Swami Janakananda, Ole Schmidt, Turiya, Maryam Abrishami and Sanna Kuittinen.

Everyone who has searched for answers to what they perceived through an activated ajna chakra. In yoga, they have learned the principles behind the universe, the collective consciousness, and the creative power, Kundalini Shakti. The duality behind everything, both what we see and what we do not see. Together we help to pass on the previous secret knowledge, about our gunas, nadis, and chakras, to anyone who wants to be seen.

THE AUTHOR

Shreyananda Natha is the author of over twelve titles on yoga. Among other things, he has written the most comprehensive books on yoga in Swedish – Everything About Yoga and the study book The Yoga Bible. He is also a certified yoga and meditation teacher according to EYTF's international guidelines and has undergone a multi-year yoga teacher training under the leadership of Swami Omananda at Satyananda Ashram. Shreyananda Natha holds the highest initiation in the Tantric Natha Order. He travels frequently to Asia and India to improve himself, and to gain knowledge and inspiration. He has immersed himself in the tantric rituals and is known for his extensive knowledge of yoga, deep relaxation, and meditation

There is no authority that can say what yoga is. When you give yourself fully and completely, and experience yoga without limitations or doubts, when you become one with the true experience in yourself, the real encounter with yoga arises. Only then do you understand what yoga is – for you. You are no longer limited by ornament, shyness and artificial thought patterns that lie as a filter between you and the transformation. Yoga is a cultural-historical wealth that is still passed on from teacher to student and helps man to find his way back to his true nature. It opens us up and attracts awareness. It strengthens our self-esteem, and our entire person's spectrum of possibilities suddenly becomes visible to us. Yoga is not difficult. You do not have to be vegan or able to stand on your head. You just need to practice your yoga regularly and the rest will come by itself.

With all the love from the universe – Aum Shanti Shreyananda Natha.

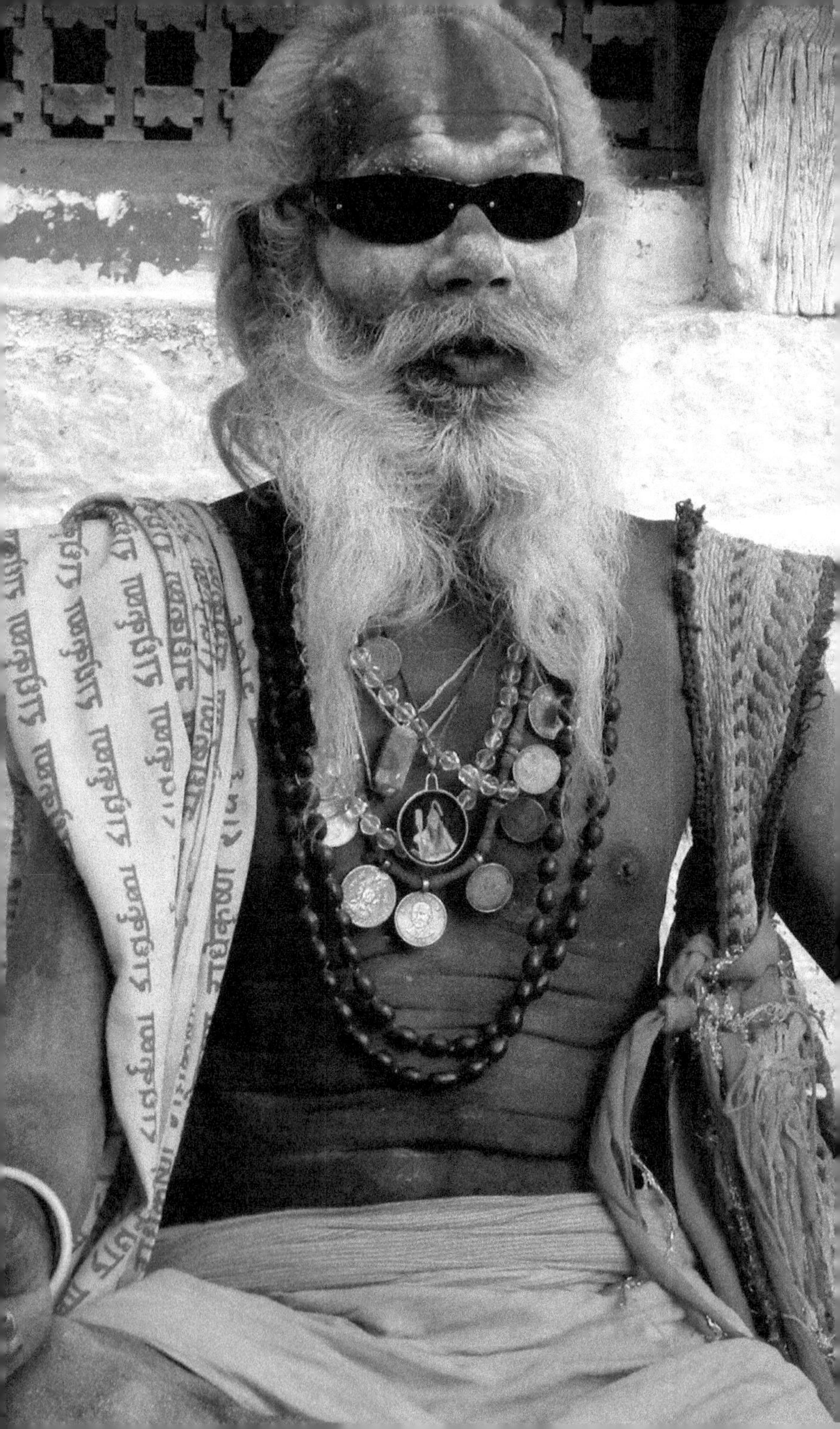

SHIVA & SHAKTI

YOGA PHILOSOPHY'S TWO PRINCIPLES: CONS-
CIOUSNESS AND ENERGY, MAN & WOMAN

CLASSICAL YOGA & ITS PHILOSOPHY

In classical yoga and its yoga philosophy, Prakriti (Shakti) is described as the cosmic energy.
It is the original essence behind everything we
can experience, both rough and subtle. Prakriti
is not in solid form, there is nothing that can be
"touched". Prakriti acts as a tool for Purusha
(Shiva). Our mind is a result of Prakriti. In order
for consciousness to be able to experience and
expand and experience itself, Prakriti is needed.
Without Prakriti, consciousness cannot become
self-aware.

The qualities of Prakritis are what build up our
bodies and our world. They carry karma and
samskaras through which living beings come
into existence and which also shape our senses.
Prakriti consists of three qualities: sattva, rajas
and tamas. These three qualities are a basis for
the other elements.

PRAKRITI, PURUSHA
All experiences. The experience.

Manifested. Unmanifest.

Background to everything. Eternal subject.

Materially and mentally. Infinite amount.

THREE PRINCIPLES BUILD A COSMOS
It is thus from these three principles that our
whole world is built – in varying combinations
of rajas, tamas and sattva. The cosmos, society and every human being are governed by the
interactions between these gunas.

There are two basic "laws" that describe how
the interaction between these three works. The
first is the "law of alternation", which means
that they are in constant motion and in collabo-
ration with each other. In sattva, rajas and tamas also exist; in rajas, tamas and sattva exist;
and in tamas, rajas and sattva exist. They work
together all the time.

The second is the "law of continuity". This
means that when a guna has become dominant,
it tends to be so for some time to come.

In yoga, a sattvic state is seen as something of a higher quality, the state that causes us to develop spiritually. Yoga practice consists of two steps: to develop a sattvic condition and to then go beyond this condition. This means that we should first purify the body and mind and then go beyond the body and mind and experience what is our true nature beyond all manifestation. There is also a hidden, mysterious knowledge tradition about activating our chakra system that we will go through later. The basic precondition for the chakra system to be activated is that the sushumna is open, and that is when we are in a sattvic state.

In scientific terms, these three gunas are described as:

SATTVA: Pure vibration / balanced

RAJAS: Movement

TAMAS: Inertia / slow / immobility

We talk about three human characters. The guna that dominates us determines what character we have. We should know the different personality traits and adapt the yoga practice accordingly.

If we are tamasic or slow, this works with a dynamic form of yoga where we get activity going in the body and in this way can create balance. Hatha yoga or physical work suits people who are tamasic.

If we are rajasic or mobile, we often have difficulty concentrating. In this case it is important to include a lot of relaxation, but to be able to relax and release tension, a dynamic form of yoga is also required. We exhaust our body and mind to then be able to relax more easily. Hatha yoga, bhakti yoga (for example, kirtan), japa yoga and karma yoga are suitable for people who are rajasic.

If we are sattvic or balanced, it is already easy to focus and concentrate and this state is well suited to satsang and studies. But even if we are sattvic, we need to work with the body. This is to create balance to the already balanced thought activities.

A rule to follow is that inertia is balanced with

movement, and movement is balanced with even more movement. We always start with the outer, the surface – our body – and go inward, deeper: we always balance and activate.

ISHWARA

Yoga is a practical method based on the samkhya philosophy, but unlike samkhya, yoga's view of creation is theistic.

In classical yoga, the God or creator is called Ishwara in Sanskrit. Ishvara is said to be the force that creates, maintains and destroys the world through the three forms Brahma, Vishnu and Shiva, as well as their female counterparts Saraswathi, Lakshmi and Kali.

Although Ishvara is very similar to the monotheistic conception of God, it differs in that Ishvara works through different gods and goddesses, and it has different shapes and manifestations. Ishwara can also be worshipped in a female form and is then called Ishwari. This is common in many yoga traditions and especially those of tantric origin. Ishwari is then equated with Shakti.

Ishvara is not described separately in samkhya, but in many yoga traditions Ishvara is described as Purusha (Shiva in tantrism).

DARSHANS

Vedas are writings composed of rishis (sight / medium) and yogis about 5,000 years ago (they can also be much older). These describe the wisdom behind the cosmic mind, which is said to be the origin of the universe and creation. These writings have from the beginning been passed on orally and then been written down. Yoga has its roots in Vedic teachings. Rishis gave Vedic knowledge a practical form, yoga.

From the Vedas, six philosophical paths or views were developed, the shad darshans, meaning "six ways of seeing" or "six ways of insight". Classical yoga as described by Patanjali in the Yoga Sutras is one of these.

Hiranyagarbha, the sun god and the cosmic creator, is traditionally said to be the creator of the yoga system.

The six Vedic / spiritual paths:

1. Nyaya – logical doctrine – Gautama.
2. Vaisheshika – atomic doctrine – Kannada.
3. Samkhya – the doctrine of the cosmic principle – Kapila.
4. Yoga – the doctrine of yoga – Hiranyagarbha.
5. Purva mimamsa / vedanta – ritual doctrine – Jaimini.
6. Yttara mimamsa / vedanta – theological doctrine – Badarayana.

Nayaya and vaisheshka are teachings based on logical philosophy. These can be compared to Plato's philosophy as we know it in the West.

Samkhya is the philosophy behind yoga and ayurveda. It is based on a scientific approach that explores both our inner and outer reality. Samkhya describes tattwas, or cosmic principles, that one tries to gain insight into and experience with the help of various yogic exercises. Samkhya describes the knowledge behind the different elements and yoga is a technique that should purify and balance the corresponding elements in ourselves.

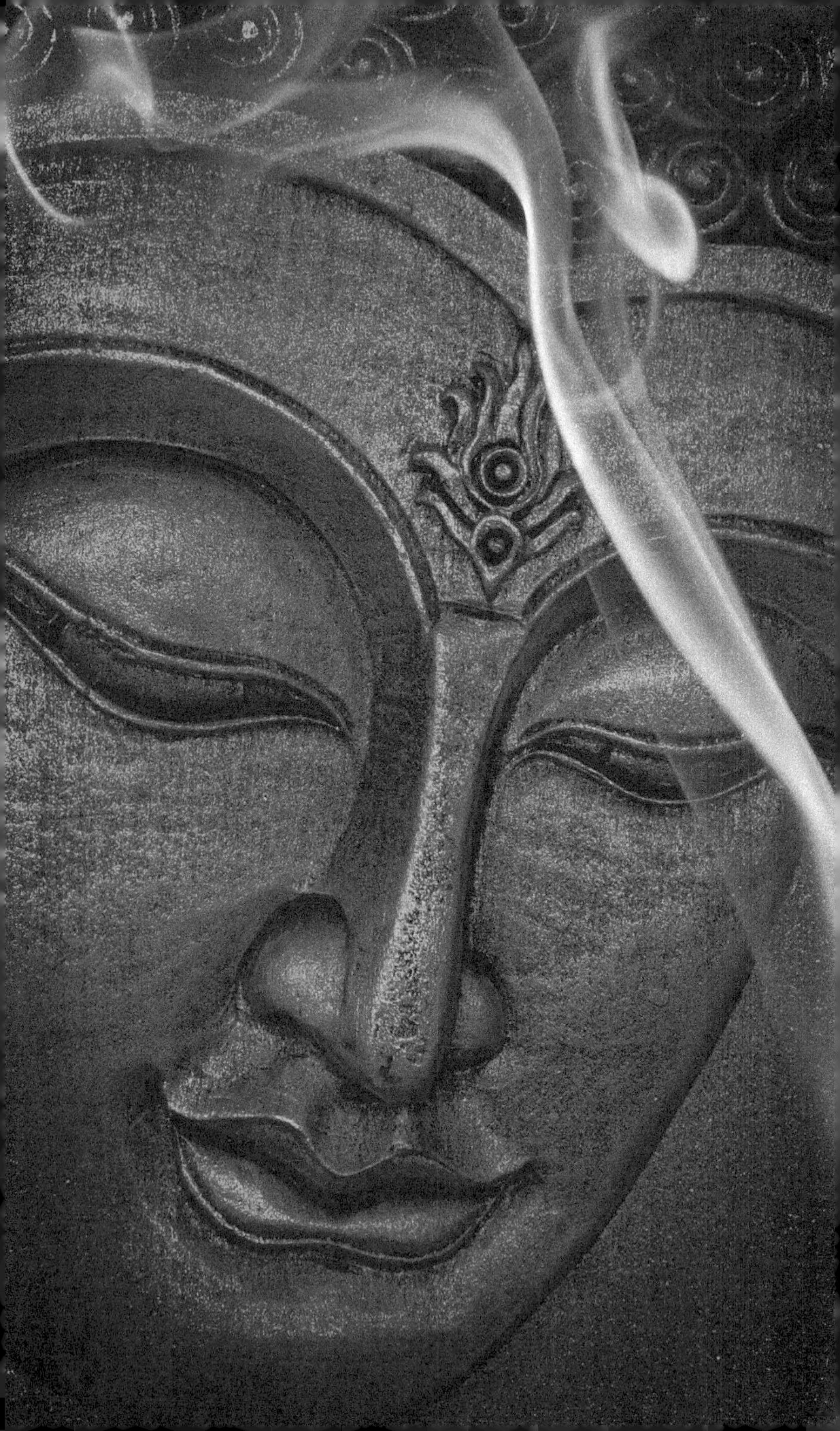

Purva mimamsa refers to karma yoga where it acts as a channel for the creative energy of the universe. We contribute to people and society with selfless services and work. It is also part of focusing on a prayer or a mantra during the work. This cleanses both the mind and the body and is a good preparation for meditation.

Uttara mimamsa is the system where we go in depth into the Vedic texts. We discuss God, the soul, the absolute and their interaction with each other.

AUM

A common symbol in yoga is Om. The symbol is made up of three syllables that together form a whole. In Sanskrit, the vowel "o" consists of "a + u". So Om can also be spelled as Aum. It represents the trinity of our existence.

The symbol A–u–m consists of three "curves", a semicircle and a point. The largest "curve" that is also at the bottom refers to our waking state when our consciousness is turned outwards and when we take in the environment with the help of our sense organs. It's called jagarat. That it is symbolised by the largest "curve" is due to the fact that it is the most common state we are in. Beta waves dominate in this state – we are aware.

The second largest curve that is autumn on the symbol refers to deep sleep and our unconscious state. We neither dream nor feel desire. This condition is called sushputi. Delta waves dominate in this state – we are unconscious.

The smallest curve that is between these two refers to our dream state, swapana. Here the consciousness is turned inwards, we experience the world with closed eyes. Theta waves dominate in this state. The experience of the subconscious.

The point in the symbol refers to our fourth state of consciousness which in Sanskrit is called turiya. Here we look neither outwards nor inwards but are in pure being. That is the unmanifest the state of Purusha. Alpha waves dominate in this state – we are super conscious.

The semicircle refers to the maya, which separates the point turiya from the "three curves". Maya symbolises what hinders our ability to experience our true nature. The semicircle tells us that maya cannot change the true experience that exists within us, the stillness / being / bliss. Maya can only master what is manifested.

Aum thus symbolises the manifested and the unmanifested – what we can see and what we cannot see – and represents the trinity of our existence. The sound and vibrations that occur when we sound Om / Aum affect our whole being on all these levels and are a very strong mantra. They permeate our entire interior and make us vibrate in step with the universe. Aum – the sound / vibration of the universe and creation.

VIVEKA

Patanjali (the author of the Yoga Sutra) describes something called viveka, that is, discernment. The purpose of eight-step yoga (the classical form of yoga) is precisely to develop viveka within us; that is, awareness, which is a prerequisite for understanding the purpose of yoga.

It requires a sharp ability to pay attention and be able to distinguish the experiencer from the experience, to see what is our true identity and

what is perishable. We also need sharp attention to understand the reasons for our ignorance
of this distinction; those include mistaking what
is changeable for immutable; mistaking what
is destructive for edification; mistaking desires
for need, and identifying with the ego instead of
the true self.

VAIRAGYA

When we have developed viveka, a change takes
place with us. We begin to let go of our desires.
This is called vairagya. We no longer cling to
what will disappear anyway. When we understand the principle of transience, we can take a
more understanding approach to life's worries
and troubles. If you read about the yoga philosophy, you understand that Buddha was enlightened in India about the same time as Patanjali
where he took his inspiration for the eightfold
path. People often talk about Buddhism as a
cousin of the yoga philosophy. Many of the ideas
are similar.

RAGA

Everything that we experience and "take in"
from our surroundings happens with our senses,
through our eyes (sight), ears (hearing), nose

(scent), tongue (taste), body / skin (feeling),
mind (thoughts, feelings, images). They can
then be divided into comfortable, uncomfortable
and neutral experiences. Most often we want to
relive the experiences that are comfortable and
provide enjoyment. We want to recreate these
experiences time and time again. This is called
raga.

Events that we experience as painful and un-
pleasant, we want to avoid. Most of the time
we try to find what gives us pleasure and avoid
what is painful. This creates dissatisfaction and
a divided mind. We do not feel satisfied with
what is. We do not accept life for what it is.

DRASHTA BHAVA

In yoga, we try to create a third approach called
drashta bhava. This can be translated as "witness attitude". Here we try to have a neutral
and relaxed attitude to our thoughts, both nega-
tive and positive. This approach, together with
viveka, leads to liberation, the ultimate purpose of yoga. To be free from desire, not to be
controlled by thoughts and feelings. To be happy
with what is – right now, whatever it looks like.
To accept what we cannot change.

SATYANANDA YOGA

Today, classical yoga is taught through, among other things, Satyananda yoga. This is a system developed by Swami Satyananda Saraswati in which they use ancient and traditional techniques: asanas to create balance between body and mind, pranayamas to work with the energy body, and meditation to calm and focus the mind. Tradition also teaches the yogic lifestyle in general to both the "ordinary modern man" and the more devoted practitioner. Everyone can take part in yoga. Jnana, bhakti and karma yoga, among others, are also part of the Satyananda system.

In Satyananda yoga, we take into account the whole being of man, not just the body. We want to give the individual an opportunity to discover and develop all aspects of their personality with the help of yoga. It is believed that change is something that happens with regular practice, under full presence and awareness. Not by pushing the body or mind beyond its means.

SRI SWAMI SIVANANDA SARASWATI

Swami Satyananda's guru and perhaps India's

most famous yoga personality, Sri Swami
Sivananda Saraswati, was born in Pattamadai
in 1887. Sivananda worked as a doctor before
giving up his job to find his guru in the Hima-
layas. He settled in Rishikesh where he was
initiated into dashnami sannyasa by his guru
Swami Vishwananda Saraswati in 1924. Over
the years, he and his disciples wrote hundreds
of books and articles on yoga and spirituality to
spread the knowledge to the general public. Sri
Swami Sivananda wanted to give the needy the
knowledge that could help them, whether it was
about improving physical health, creating peace
of mind or developing spiritually. This still cha-
racterises Satyananda yoga today.

SWAMI SATYANANDA SARASWATI

Swami Satyananda Saraswati was born in Al-
mora in 1923. At the age of nineteen, he met
Sukhman Giri from Juna-Akhara, a tantric yogini
from Nepal. From her he learned, among other
things, the new tantric nyasa techniques, which
he developed further with Swami Sivananda.
Nyasa are techniques for raising awareness by
placing different energies in the body parts.
From these he then developed the world-famous
deep relaxation yoga nidra. In 1943 he then met

his guru Swami Sivananda and was initiated into dashnami sannyasa in 1947. After serving his guru's mission for twelve years, Satyananda began his journey through India as an ascetic to discover the needs of society. In 1956, Swami Satyananda founded the International Yoga Fellowship and in 1963 the Bihar School of Yoga, hoping to spread ancient yogic knowledge to all corners of the world. For twenty years, Swami Satyananda then travelled around the world, spreading the knowledge of yoga. He and his disciples also authored over eighty books on yoga, tantra and spirituality. In 1984, he founded the Yoga Research Foundation and Sivananda Math to help those who were disadvantaged in society.

"I'M WAITING TO LEAVE THIS BODY, BUT I'M NOT GOING TO LEAVE IT UNTIL I GET MY RETURN TICKET. I DO NOT WANT EMANCIPATION, MOKSHA, OR ANY PERSONAL SATISFACTION WHICH COMES WITH SPIRITUAL ENLIGHTENMENT. MY AIM AND ASPIRATION IN THIS AND IN ALL FUTURE LIVES IS TO HELP OTHERS. TO WIPE THE TEARS OF SUFFERING AND PAIN FROM THE EYES OF EVERY PERSON WHO IS SEEKING SOLACE, PEACE, PLENTY AND PROSPERITY. THAT IS THE ONLY PURPOSE OF MY LIFE"

(SWAMI SATYANANDA SARASWATI)

YOGA FORMS

In Satyananda yoga, the following forms of yoga are applied:

JNANA YOGA

The path of spiritual insight where we, through intellectual and theoretical knowledge, study life and try to distinguish the true from the perishable. This path is suitable for people who are theoretically inclined.

BHAKTI YOGA

The path of devotion and love which consists of song and dance or meditation on an image of a guru or the divine. The practitioner strives to create a personal relationship with the divine and merge with it.

KARMA YOGA

Selfless service where we help other people and society without taking advantage of it or shining in the glory.

HATHA YOGA

Here we want to balance and strengthen the physical and mental body as a preparation for the more advanced exercises in kundalini yoga.

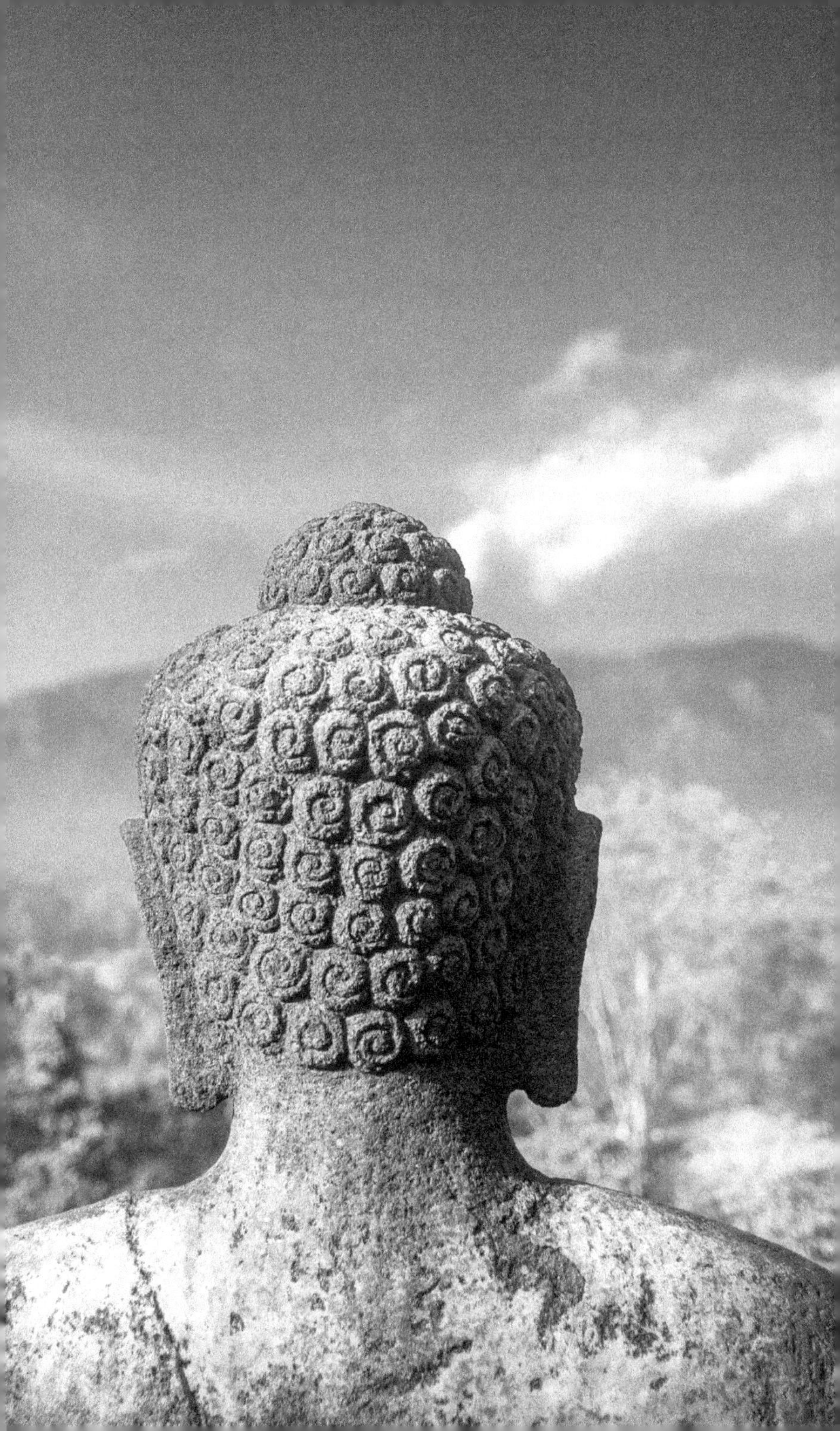

Asanas, pranayamas, bandhas and shatkarmas are used.

RAJA YOGA – CLASSIC YOGA

The path of meditation. This refers to the system described in Patanjali's Yoga Sutras.

KRIYA YOGA

Satyananda taught kriya yoga based on the secret exercises of yoga and tantra shastras. Kriya means "activity" or "movement" and refers to the natural movement of consciousness. Kriya yoga does not stop the movements of the mind but instead creates an activity in the mind that leads to a conscious increase and to awakening. There are seventy kriyas, of which twenty are best known and used.

THE TRADITIONS

In addition to the yogic tradition, Satyananda yoga also includes the tantric and Vedic traditions.

Tantra refers to practical exercises which lead to the expansion of the human consciousness and the awakening of kundalini Shakti. The principle behind the tantric system is that one uses the material world and experiences of it to become enlightened.

Tantra is often described as a sexual tradition where practitioners want to enhance the sexual experience. Originally, tantra was intended to awaken kundalini Shakti, which is a dormant potential force in people.

There are many tantric paths and the common denominator of these paths is the use of mantras, yantras (concentration symbols used to liberate consciousness), chakras, mandalas (discovering macrocosm in microcosm), tapasya (self-purification), raja yoga, pranayama, shaktipat (power transmission) and tantric initiations to reach awakening.

Tantrism advocates a life in which the qualities of the intellect and the heart are exploited. The aim is to be able to discern and focus with the help of the intellect and to be able to see and experience with the heart the unseen, the cosmic consciousness beyond the material.

The Vedic tradition is one of the oldest-preserved spiritual traditions in existence. It advocates the divine as the ultimate truth and a life accordingly in the material world.

Central to Vedic doctrine is that God is constantly present, omniscient and omnipotent while the individual is only an actor. In order to experience the reality that is satyam (truth), shivam (favourable) and sundaram (beautiful), the individual should live a life where they strive to harmonise thoughts, behaviour and actions.

A meditative contemplation; belief in God and oneself; living in harmony with, and being grateful for, the environment and nature; and experiencing unity are the foundations of the Vedic tradition.

All the Vedic and tantric traditions are held together by yoga. Yoga is the practical principle of the spiritual paths that leads to an increased awareness and self-insight.

RAJA YOGA: THE ROYAL PATH

Patanjali never gave his system any specific title. He simply called it yoga. In time, however, his method became known as Patanjali's yoga and or classical yoga. Patanjali's yoga is one

of the different forms of raja yoga (raja means
royal) that also include:

Kundalini yoga (also called Laya yoga)
Kriya yoga
Yoga mantra
Dhyana yoga
Patanjali yoga

Raja yoga is the doctrine of the mind. Here
we explore our inner world to be able to take
advantage of our strength and knowledge. Raja
yoga teaches different methods to create a focused mind. It is based on mental discipline.

Patanjali himself defined his method as "elimination of mental fluctuations", usually translated to "when the mind is still, yoga occurs". The
mind can be described as the visible part of the
pure consciousness and divided into the conscious, the subconscious and the unconscious.
Patanjali's definition means that "yoga is the
control of the pattern of consciousness".

VIYOGA
Who is experiencing?

Most people know that yoga means union, but in the Yoga Sutras, Patanjali describes yoga as a process of separation. This can be explained by the samkhya philosophy, which is the foundation of the Yoga Sutras.

Samkhya divides existence and individuality into two different aspects that we have touched on before – Purusha and Prakriti. Existence and the individual are created when these two merge. Purusha refers to the one who sees / experiences, drashta. Prakriti refers to the seen, drishya.

Practicing yoga and its process leads to viyoga, which is a separation between the one who experiences and the seen. This in turn leads to yoga, the association that is the very development of yoga, the culmination. At first Purusha and Prakriti must be separated from each other and then it is understood that these are in fact one and the same.

It can also be described that the pure consciousness (Purusha) is broken down by incorrect identification with mind and body (Prakriti). The purpose of yoga is to release the pure consciousness from the mind and body.

The experience of the difference and separation of Purusha and Prakriti leads to the realisation that everything is one and the same.

EIGHT STEPS / ASHTANGA

Patanjali describes a series of techniques that have a slow and harmonising effect on our mind and perception. The most important thing in Patanjali's system is described in the eight steps. The first five steps are preparatory to the other three steps and belong to bhairanga (outer yoga). Ashtanga means eight different steps and should not be confused in this context with the modern ashtanga yoga developed by yoga master Shri K. Pattabhi Jois.

We must not see the first five steps as a staircase; we can rather see it as a wheel whereby, working with one spoke, we also influence the others.

1. Yama – about moral discipline in social life.

2. Niyama – about restraint on a personal level.

3. Asana – sitting position / body position. This refers to the correct meditation position / lotus position so that you can remain immobile during

the meditation and are not distracted by the physical body.

4. Pranayama – respiratory regulation / control of prana / kumbhaka. By controlling breathing, you can control the life force / prana in the body and calm the mind.

5. Pratyahara – removal of sensory impressions. By blocking sensory impressions, one is not distracted by the external environment.

The last three steps belong to antharanga (inner yoga). In order to develop in depth and succeed with these steps, we must have absorbed the first five preparatory steps. The steps before pratyahara gradually dissolve our external ob-stacles while the exercises afterwards eliminate thoughts and inner images so that the mind is still. Ida (our inner world) becomes balanced with pingala (our outer world) so that the sus-humna (our supersensible world) begins to exist during samadhi.

6. Dharana – concentration. Focus on a medita-tion object.

7. Dhyana – meditation. After a longer period of concentration, we naturally sink into meditation. Here one is fulfilled by the meditation object.

8. Samadhi – liberation / ecstasy / superconscious. Meditation eventually leads to samadhi. Here the movements of the mind have stopped and we become one with the meditation object and experience powerful ecstasy / joy. There are twelve stages of samadhi where the last stage leads to the liberation of the cycle of rebirths.

The eight steps gradually balance our five koshas (shells): annamaya, pranamaya, manomaya, vijnamaya and anandamaya. The boundary between the shells is loosened from the coarsest, the body – annamaya kosha – to the most subtle, our innermost interior – anandamaya kosha.

YAMA

Satya – truth, to be true to oneself and others.
Ahimsa – do not be involved in killing.
Asteya – do not steal, not to take more than you need and to share.
Aparighara – not to be greedy, to live in material simplicity.

Brahmacharya – chastity. To live ascetically, not
to indulge in pleasures, as they are considered
to distract one from reaching the goal of yoga.

NIYAMA

Saucha – purity of speech and action, sensory
impressions (media, television, radio), food,
hygiene.
Santosha – contentment, to be happy with what
you have. If we focus on what we do not have,
we create even more emptiness within ourselves. If we focus on shortages, we get even more
shortages (the law of attraction).
Tapas – self-discipline, hardening of the inner
fire.
Swadhyaya – studies.
Ishwara pranidhara – to surrender one's personal will to the higher will.

Yamas thus create a balance in our interaction
with the outside world and niyamas harmonise
our inner feelings. These rules are created to
balance our external actions with our internal
settings. The mind affects our external actions
at the same time as our external actions affect
the mind. If our actions are not good, the mind
will also be negatively affected, which creates a

vicious circle, as a distracted mind creates less good actions. Yamas and niyamas are designed to break the vicious cycle. It can be difficult to follow these rules in full, but even a small change does a lot to balance the mind.

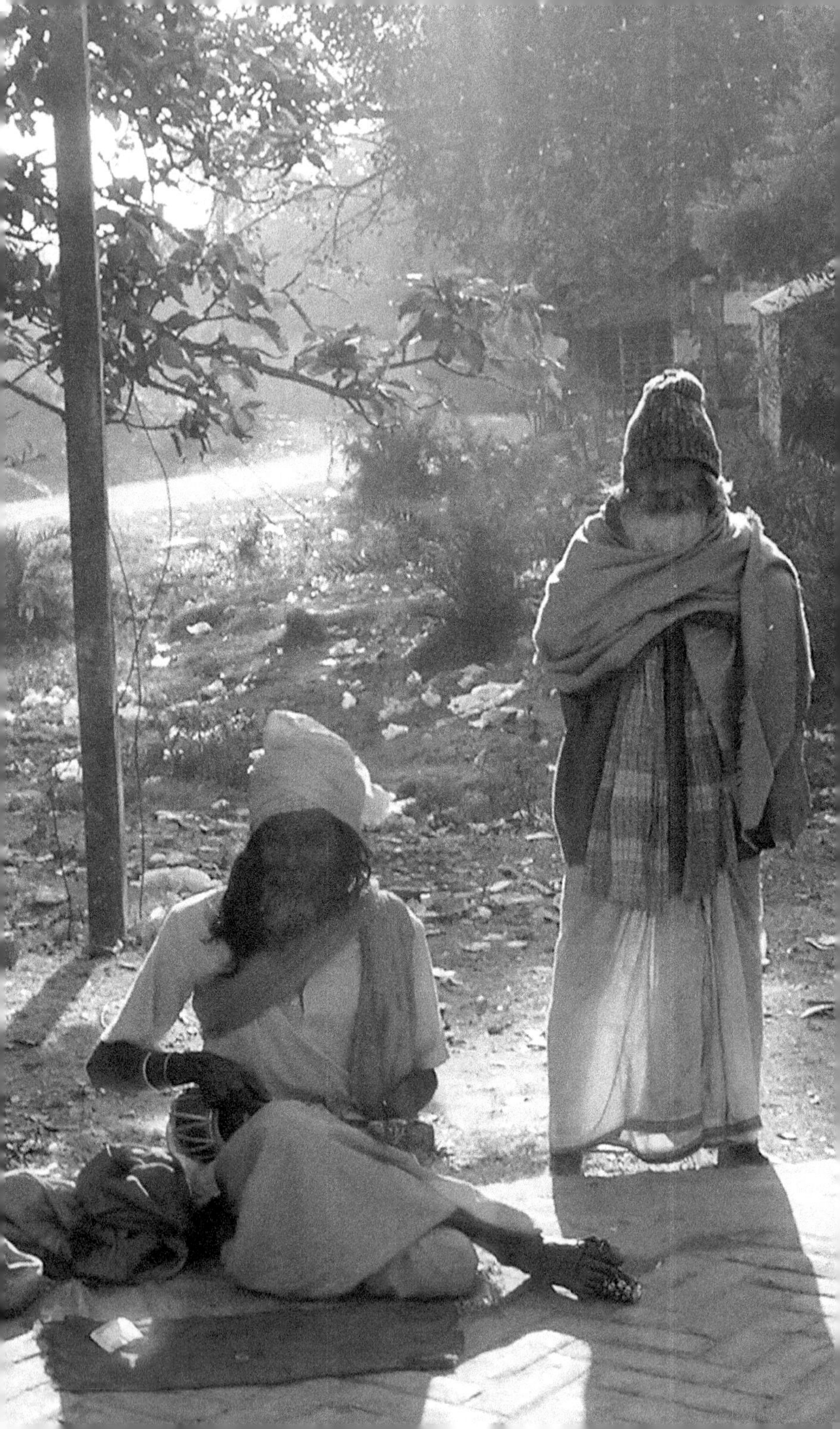

PATANJALIS YOGA SUTRAS

Patanjali's work consists of 196 sutras. The word sutra itself is often incorrectly translated as verse. The actual translation is "to thread", which also describes how the sutras are linked to each other and carry an underlying continuity. The work is seen as the most accurate and scientific yogic text ever written down.

Who Patanjali was and when he lived is still unclear. It has also not been possible to determine when his work was written and whether he really was a man or a woman. There is still some evidence that he must have lived around 300 to 400 BCE.

Patanjali gives us a range of techniques that gradually balance and harmonise our mind. The unique thing is that Patanjali does not describe a single yoga position in the way we are usually used to. Here, instead, the focus is on yoga from a moral perspective. When Patanjali talked about asana, he referred to a steady and comfortable position to sit and meditate in.

Many great masters and yogis have translated and interpreted Patanjali's work.

The following sutras are some of the most important to know. They are the essence of the practice.

3: 2
CAUSE OF SUFFERING.

Avidyāsmitārāgadveṣābhiniveśāh kleśāh

Avidy: erroneous knowledge, asmit: I-experience, raga: liking, dves: reluctance, abhiniveh: fear of death, klesah: suffering.

Klesha is the suffering that is present in everyone. The basis of all suffering according to Patanjali is incorrect identification with the experience. Everyone carries a subconscious suffering but we are seldom aware of it as our daily life, all the musts and chores block the experience of it.

We rarely become aware of our fear of dying, even if it is in our subconscious. The fear of dying is the basis of our greatest suffering.

Kleshas are like a chain of misfortune that begins with our ignorance of our true nature based on our ego. We try to find pleasure and avoid suffering, which in turn creates fear and tension. The solution to being free from suffering is meditation.

4: 2
THE ROOT CAUSE.

Avidyākṣetramuttareṣām prasuptatanuvichchhinnodārāṇām

Avidya: incorrect knowledge, ksetram: area, uttaresam: of the following, prasupta: dormant, tanu: weak, vichchhinna: alternating, udaranam: fully active.

Avidya is the field of dormant, weak, alternating and fully active states of kleshas.

Avidya is the basis of the other four kleshas: asmita, raga, dweshta and abhinivesha. These are either dormant, weak, alternating or fully active in nature. When we learn to deal with avidya, we can also more easily learn to deal with the other four kleshas.

Avidya is about the ignorance of our true nature.
In order to find our way back to our true nature,
we must learn to control the kleshas.

5: 2
INCORRECT KNOWLEDGE.

**Anityāśuchiduhkhānātmasu nityaśuchisukhātmak-
hyātiravidyā**

Anitya: not eternal, asuchi: unclean, duhkha:
pain, natmasu: not atman, nitya: eternal, suchi:
pure, sukha: goodness, atma: self, khyati:
knowledge, avidya: erroneous knowledge.

Avidya means that one confuses the eternal,
impure and evil with the eternal, pure, good and
atman.

Avidaya is about ignorance of our true nature
and about our identification with the body.
We are free from avidaya by developing our
discernment, viveka. Through viveka we can
distinguish between our body and atman, our
inner true self.

Avidaya is also called maya. In a cosmic context

it is called maya and on an individual level it is
called avidaya.

6: 2
SEPARATION, I, EGO.

Dṛgdarśanaśaktyorekātmatevāsmitā

Drg: Purusha, the power of consciousness, dars-
ana: the seen, saktyoh: of the two forces, ekat-
mate: identity, eva: like that, dodge: I-feeling.

Asmita can be described as an identification of
Purusha as a buddhi.

Asmita means that our inner consciousness, our
true self is mixed with our existence, body, actions and mind. When our true self is expressed
through the body, actions and mind, it is called
asmita. Purusha is identified by its means of
expression / instrument.

This can be expressed in different ways: as
identification with the body or in a more intel-
lectually developed person as identification with
the more developed sensory functions.

Our ability to see, think and hear comes from Purusha, which is expressed through our senses. When we mix these together it is called asmita.

It is Shakti, the power of Purusha that lies behind the ability to think, see, etc. which is mixed with the actual means / instrument with which these are expressed.

By meditating, we can come to the realisation that Purusha is not a part of the body or the intellect (buddhi). We come across asmita.

7: 2
ATTRACTION, I WANT.

Sukhānuśayå rāgah

Sukha: satisfaction, anusayl: accompanying, ragah: pleasure, liking.

Raga is the pleasure created by satisfaction.

Raga is about the mind constantly wanting to recreate a previous experience of pleasure.

8: 2

REPULSION, I DO NOT WANT.

Duhkahānuśayå dveṣah

Duhka: pain, anusayl: accompanying, dvesah: reluctance.

Dwesha is our reluctance to experience pain.

Dwesha is the opposite of raga. You want to avoid what creates discomfort. Raga and dwesha keep us in the lower stages of consciousness. As long as raga and dwesha are allowed to rule over us, we do not develop spiritually.

To like something also means that you do not like the opposite of what you like. So raga and dwesha are not really opposites, but two sides of the mind. Dwesha is what affects us most negatively because it is based on hatred. Elimination of dweshta allows for a deeper meditation and a natural elimination of raga.

9: 2

FEAR OF DYING.

Svarasavāhī viduṣo ´pi tathārūdho ´bhiniveśah

Svarasavahi: persistence of self, vidusah: of the learned, api: also, tatha: like it, rudhah: dominant, abhinivesah: fear of death.

Abnivecha is the hope of being able to live and be maintained by one's own power even among the scholars.

This is the most dominant klesha. Fear of dying is experienced by all individuals. It is an innate inherent force that exists naturally in us, a self-preservation drive. As children, we do not experience this in the same way, but the older we get, the more aware we become of it.

In those who have developed viveka, abhinivecha is almost eliminated, but in most people it can be seen in its most active form, which can also lead to fear and panic in, for example, a serious illness. In ancient Indian texts one can read about the cause of abhnivecha, which is said to be the identification with the body.

11: 2

MEDITATION - THE SOLUTION TO THE ELIMINATION OF KLESHAS.

45

Dhyānaheyāstadvṛttayah

Dhyana: meditation, heyah: reduces, tadvrttay-ah: modification, change.

The modification of the kleshas can be reduced through meditation.

We can learn to understand our fears / kles-has by observing the mind. These exist in our subconscious as well as in our conscious mind to varying degrees. In our normal daily state, we rarely see the character of the kleshas. We can not eliminate the kleshas with the help of the intellect, it can only be done with the help of meditation.

It takes a sharp ability to pay attention to beco-me aware of how kleshas look in ourselves. For example, we may believe that we are not afraid of death even though we unconsciously are. We do not see it. Even individuals who have been engaged in spiritual development for a long time

– who for several years have experienced peace and have thought they are free samskaras and kleshas – can suddenly experience obstacles and failure. The seed, root and cause of the kleshas remain and come up to the surface.

To get rid of kleshas in depth, you need to practice the whole system of yoga: yamas, niyamas and kriya yoga.

By dhyana, we mean to observe what happens to us mentally. This is done by paying attention to our thoughts, both good and bad, and by letting them come to the surface. In the long run, it prevents kleshas from manifesting in the most active form, which creates suffering and fear in our daily lives. In this case, one does not refer to "object focus" when talking about dhyana but to assume mouna, that is, focusing on how kleshas look and their character and strength.

By focusing and observing, vrittis is weakened. This explains why meditation has such a calming effect on us. During meditation, our unconscious fears can come to the surface so that we become aware of them. Tensions caused by our fears / kleshas are weakened and we can relax. A feeling of inner harmony arises.

When our fears (kleshas) have taken on a more latent form, we should, through our discernment (viveka), try to find the cause of the fear. Maybe we are dependent on something or maybe we want to be successful.

Dhyana (raja yoga) and viveka (jnana yoga) are thus two important tools in the elimination of our fears (kleshas). To prevent being drawn back to the unconscious state again – where our experiences risk becoming too difficult to deal with, karma yoga and bhakti yoga can be very helpful.

"A MAN WHO IS AFRAID OF DEATH WILL
BE AFRAID OF LIFE ALSO, BECAUSE LIFE
BRINGS DEATH. IF YOU ARE AFRAID OF
THE ENEMY AND YOU CLOSE THE DOOR,
THE FRIEND WILL ALSO BE PROHIBITED."

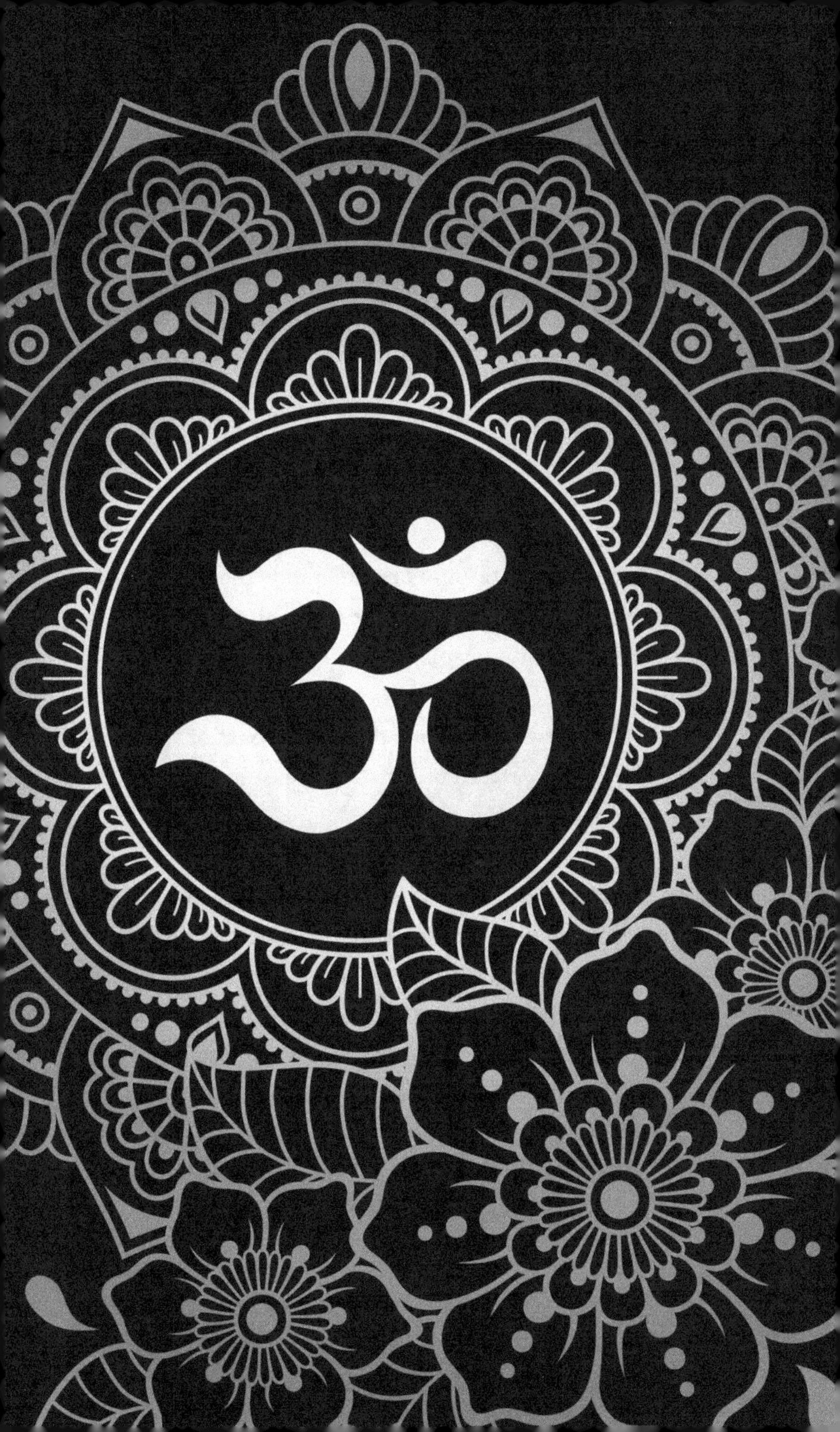

2: 1

WHAT IS YOGA?

Yogaschitta vṛitti nirodhah

Yogah: yoga, chitta: consciousness, vritti: patterns, movements, nirodhah: blocked – still.
When the movements of the mind are still, yoga
occurs.

The term chitta refers to the mind, the individual consciousness on the conscious, unconscious
and subconscious plane.

Nirodhah aims to block the movements of the
mind, the pattern of consciousness, not the
mind or consciousness itself.

This happens automatically when we sleep.
The normal flow of vrittis is stopped and we
are moved to another state of consciousness.
We experience other things, people, events and
places. From this we can understand that within
us there is something that exists independently
of our body, mind and life energy (prana), something that is something completely different
than any of these. This "something" is consci

ousness, a constant and uninterrupted state of consciousness.

Vritti can be translated as "circular" and this describes what chitta's movements look like. They are like rings on the water.

So, what is yoga? Yoga is to calm the movements of the mind on all planes of consciousness. It is not about shutting down or trying to shield oneself from the external impressions that we encounter every day. What we want is to get past the experiences and visions that our individual consciousness creates during deep meditation and higher stages of samadhi. When this happens, yoga occurs. This is a prerequisite for the development of human consciousness.

When one ceases to identify with Prakriti, the three gunas develop our consciousness.

People talk about the five different characters of the mind. If you compare these with the kundalini awakening, you can see that moodha (the sluggish mind) is associated with mooladhara chakra where the individual consciousness is dormant.

After a period of practicing specific exercises, the consciousness is stimulated so that it directs itself to the area around the navel, manipura chakra. This state of consciousness is called kshipta and belongs to rajas. Most often, however, it sinks down to mooladhara chakra again and then rises to swadhisthana chakra, manipura chakra and again to mooladhara chakra. Once consciousness has stabilised in the manipura chakra for some time – vikshipta – it will steer further through the anahata chakra and the vishuddhi chakra to the ajna chakra. In this state of consciousness, ekagrata, the consciousness is completely focused and concentrated, sattvic. Further in the sahasrara chakra one achieves the state of nirodha which is beyond the three gunas and then also sattvic.

All functions in our body, mind and environment are governed by the interaction between the three gunas. Even though one guna dominates, the other two are present all the time and affect our conscious state. We should learn to see which guna dominates and how the other two come into play and then learn to balance these in order to be able to control consciousness.

3: 1

WHEN YOGA CULMINATES - THEN THE SIGHT IS ESTABLISHED.

53

Tadā draṣṭuh svarūpe´vasthānam

Tada: then, drasuh: seeing – answer, upe: the basic nature of oneself, vasthanam: establish, develop.

The seeing develops in its own true nature.

Self-awareness, kaivalya, is the very goal of yoga in this context. It develops when the activity of chitta vritti ceases, when the mind is no longer affected by the interaction of the three gunas and when one ceases to identify with the material world.

The insight into our true nature comes from within. It is not possible to create or experience this insight in the state of consciousness where one still identifies with the self, the ego. It takes a purity of mind, complete mind control and freedom from desire to be able to reach this insight.

4: 1

WHAT ELSE HAPPENS TO PURUSHA?

Vátti sārūpyamitaratra

Vrtti: modification, pattern, sarupyam: identification, itaratra: other state.

Otherwise there is an identification with the movements of the mind.

When the movements of the mind, chitta vrittis, are not in the state of nirodha – have not calmed down – Purusha can not become aware of himself. Instead, there is an identification with chitta and its fluctuations.

When there is no awareness of the pure consciousness, Purusha, we identify with the movements of the chitta and are controlled by emotions such as feeling angry, sad or scared.

Patanjali describes different techniques that are adapted to the different needs of individuals, depending on temperament, to lead chitta to the state of nirodha. It is a prerequisite for Purusha to become aware of its true nature.

5: 1
VRITTIS - MAIN DIVISIONS.

Vṛttayah pañchatayyah kliṣṭāakliṣṭāh

Vrttayah: modification of the mind, pañchatayyah: fivefold, klista: painful, difficult, aklistah:
not painful.

The modification of the mind is fivefold, these
are either painful or not.

There are five types of vrittis and these are
either painful or non-painful. In total, there
are ten types of vrittis. When you experience
something as pleasant, for example, when you
look at a beautiful flower, it is called aklishta.
When you experience something that is painful
and uncomfortable, it is called klishta.

According to Patanjali, everything we see,
hear, think and feel are different formations
of the mind. According to the yogic system, all
our thoughts, knowledge and various planes
of consciousness are twisted, as well as our
dreams.

6: 1

FIVE TYPES OF VRITTIS.

Pramāṇa-viparyaya-vikalpa-nidrā smṛtayah

Pramana: right knowledge, viparyaya: wrong
knowledge, vikalpa: imagination, nidra: sleep,
smrtayah: memory.

The five different patterns of the mind are right
knowledge, wrong knowledge, imagination,
sleep and memory.

Our mind is made up of five different types of
vrittis; correct knowledge, false knowledge,
imagination, deep sleep and memory. These five
build up the mind and shape the three dimensi-
ons of the individual consciousness. All states of
mind belong to these five types of sensory patterns or twists (wakefulness, dreams, seeing,
speaking, hearing, touching, crying, feeling and
doing).

The ultimate goal of yoga is to break down these
manifestations of the pattern of consciousness,
that is, the vrittis.

12: 1

The importance of abhyasa and vairagya.

57

Abhyāsavairāgyābhyām tannirodhah

Abhyasa: continuous practice, vairagyabhyam: through, vairagya, tat: it, nirodhah: stills.

Calming the five movement patterns of the mind takes place through regular exercise and vairagya.

Patanjali describes two ways to stop the flow of chitta vrittis. Abhyasa and vairagya. Abhyasa means regular exercise. Vairagya aims at liberation from raga and dweshta, that is, attraction and reluctance to like / dislike. If you have control over these, meditation will be easier.

15: 1

A lower state of vairagya.

Dṛṣṭānuśravika-viṣayāvitṛṣṇasya vaśīkāra-sañjñā vairāgyam

Drsta: the seen, anusravika: the heard, visaya:

object, vitrsnasya: of the one who is free from
desire, vasikara: control, sañjña: consciousness, vairagyam: absence of desire.

The state of consciousness when the individual
becomes free from the desire to satisfy the mind
with what has previously been experienced and
what one has heard of is vairagya.

When we are free from desire, when we no
longer yearn for pleasures that we have experienced in life, it is called vairagya. We are
free from desire in the face of all objects of the
mind.

It is possible to achieve vairagya even if we live
in everyday society, have a family and a job.
It is not necessary to give these up. However,
what we absolutely must give up completely is
raga and dweshta.

Vairagya starts from within ourselves, not
from outside. It does not matter what clothes
we wear or which people we live with. What
really matters is what kind of attitude we have
towards the events and people you meet in life.

Vairagya is divided into three stages. In the
first step, you are fully aware of the desires and
unwillingness that we carry and we work to get
over raga and dweshta. In the second stage,
some objects of raga and dweshta have been
taken over, but there is still something left.
In the third stage, the mind is completely free
from these, but they can still remain latent in
the subconscious.

16: 1
A HIGHER STATE OF VAIRAGYA.

Tatparam puruṣakhyāterguṇavaitṛṣṇyam

Tat: it, param: supreme, purusakhyateh: true
knowledge of Purusha, gunavaitrsnyam: free
from the lusts of gunas.

The highest state is when one becomes free
from the lusts of gunas with the knowledge of
Purusha.

Once one has reached this higher state of vairagya, there is no longer a need to experience
pleasure and enjoyment, acquire knowledge or
be dependent on sleep. This state of vairagya is
achieved when one becomes aware of Purusha.

21: 1

Curiosity increases power and strength.

Tåvrasamvegānāmāsannah

Those who carry a strong curiosity and desire, samvega, achieve asamprajnata samadhi soon.

One realises that everything is perishable, which is a prerequisite for wanting to seek the truth.

23: 1

The degree of curiosity and devotion to Ishwara (God).

Mṛdumadhyādhimātratvāt tato´pi viśeṣah

Mrdu: small, madhya: medium, adhimatra: strong, tvat: dependent on, tatopi: even, more than, viseah: specific.

As the desire grows in intensity from being small to becoming strong, asamprajnata samadhi can be achieved faster.

God refers to a superior spiritual consciousness. It is neither physical nor mental but only
spiritual, the highest manifested consciousness
in man.

According to Patanjali, if you find it difficult to
develop spiritually through the techniques described, you can also do so by devoting yourself
intensely to God.

28: 1
SADHANA FOR ISHVARA.

Tajjapastadarthabhāvanam

Tat: it, japa: repetition of the word, tat: it,
artha: meaning, bhavanam: fill the mind.

To recite Aum and fill the mind with its meaning.

What separates Ishwara and humans is that humans are the manifested state of consciousness
while Ishwara is the highest state of consciousness. The manifested condition continues to be
manifested through rebirths or incarnations and
takes shape in various bodies such as humans

and animals. When it reaches the highest stage of evolution, it takes shape in a finer and more developed body. Ishwara is beyond manifestation, of life and death and is therefore seen as the guru of the departed masters and prophets.

One cannot reach Ishwara by thinking or speaking, nor by our intellect. Thinking and experiencing are two different things. The whole Indian philosophical system is divided into tattwa chintana, reflection of the highest consciousness, and tattwa darshan, experience of the highest consciousness. India's six philosophical systems are based on tattwa chintana (knowledge). Tattwa darshan, experience, develops through yoga, bhakti, mystery and occult rituals.

Aum is like a means of expression for Ishwara, which is otherwise completely formless. This is described in yantra, mantra and tantra. These three are the expressions of the formless. Mantra is like a term in the form of sound. Pure consciousness is denoted, described in terms of the power of sound. In tantra, there is symbolism in the form of humans and animals. Yantra is a mental symbol. Aum is both a mantra and a yantra. It is not tantra as it must have a human form and have no sound.

We cannot experience Ishwara with our eyes or ears, but we experience it within ourselves using a mantra. Aum denotes Ishvara.

Through a constant repetition of the word Aum – as well as dhyana about its meaning, the meditation becomes complete. Japa is not enough but must go hand in hand with meditation. Patanjali recommends that at the same time during the rehearsal of Aum one should be aware of japa and its significance. Therefore, it is important to understand the meaning of Aum. It is made up of three letters A–u–m. A relates to the world we perceive with our senses and body. U relates to the subconscious mind. M relates to the unconscious mind. By understanding this and repeating the mantra, one can change the three states of manifested consciousness, go beyond these and finally reach the fourth and mysterious stage of consciousness called turiya, that is, the unmanifest state of Purusha.

30-32: 1

OBSTACLES THAT MAY APPEAR DURING SADHANA AND HOW TO GET PAST THEM.

1. Disease
2. Lethargy
3. Well-being
4. Lack of action
5. Laziness
6. Strong desires
7. Wrong perception
8. Instability
9. Shaking
10. Pain
11. Depression

It is important to know and be prepared that difficulties and obstacles are part of the sadhana's path. When the consciousness is turned inwards, the metabolism and functions of the body change. We may fall asleep during meditation or have different perceptual experiences.

It can often seem that the practitioner does not care about their personal life, family and other chores. We may experience doubts, feel unsure if the sadhanan is the right one or if you will reach the goal at all.

To get rid of obstacles, we need to focus on one principle – a mantra or a symbol. We should therefore stick to a certain mantra or symbol and not change it. Otherwise, the obstacles will become a fact.

There is no real difference between the different symbols, but if we change the symbol, confusion is created in the mind.

33: 1
CREATING OPPOSITE VIRTUES - THE FOUR ATTITUDES.

Maitrīkarunāmuditopeksānam sukhaduhkhapunyā-punyavisayānām bhāvanātaśchittaprasādanam

Maitri: kindness, karuna: compassion, mudito: joy, upeksanam: indifference, sukha: happiness, duhkha: suffering, punya: virtue, apunya: burden, visayanam: goal, bhavanatah: attitude, chitta: mind, prasadanam: pure.

In order to concentrate the mind, it must first be purified and stilled. This is done by developing attitudes of kindness, compassion, joy and indifference and respect for individuals as

well as events that create joy, suffering, virtues
or mistakes.

These attitudes are:

1. Friendship with the happy.
2. Compassion for the unfortunate.
3. Gratitude and joy for what goes well.
4. Indifference to what goes wrong.

This creates a calm and undisturbed mind. It is
part of the nature of the mind to be drawn to
the outside world. It is not part of the nature
of the mind to look inward. When turning the
mind inward, one must first remove obstacles
and impurities. These four attitudes remove
these obstacles both on a conscious and an unconscious level.

34: 1
CONTROL OF PRANA.

Prachchhardanavidhāraṇābhyām vā prāṇasya

By prolonging and keeping the breath out, one
can control the mind.

The whole mental structure consists of four different parts. Depending on the individual's temperament, different yoga paths fit differently.

1. Karma yoga – dynamic people.
2. Bhakti yoga – emotional individuals.
3. Raya, kriya, swara yoga – psychic people.
4. Jnana yoga – intellectual persons.

We are often a mixture of all of these and can benefit from practicing all paths. We should choose a sadhana that suits us best to create as little resistance as possible along the way.

Patanjali describes pranayama and how, by keeping the breath inside and out of the body and through three locks, we can calm our mind. He describes maha bandha where we do jalandhara, uddiyana and moola bandha while keeping our breath out. If we are beginners, we can practice rechaka and kapalbhati.

With the help of these exercises, the mind is calmed.

There are also fine channels in the body called

nadis. Through these, prana, or impulses and signals, flow to and from the brain. In total, we have about seventy-two thousand different nadis.

Ida, pingala and sushuma are the three most important of all nadis, of which sushumna is the most important channel for spiritual consciousness. These three start from the mooladhara chakra and meet in the ajna chakra.

Our breathing controls our thoughts in the present, past and future. During the day, breathing alternates through the right and left nostrils. You usually breathe for one hour through the right nostril and then one hour through the left nostril and about twelve times a day through each. The left nostril is called the ida and the right the pingala. When the breathing changes from pingala to ida or from ida to pingala, the sushumna flows temporarily.

Performing heavy work is best suited when pingala nadi is flowing. When ida nadi flows, lighter work is best suited. When sushumna nadi flows, meditation is best suited. We can control the flow through the nostrils with the help of various exercises.

35: 1

PAY ATTENTION TO SENSORY EXPERIENCES.

**Viṣayavatī vā pravṛttirutpannā manasah sthitini-
bandhanī**

Visayavati: sensual, va: or, pravrttih: functio-
ning, panning: arises, manasah: of the mind,
sthiti: steadfastness, nibandhani: which binds.

The mind can be made steady by keeping it active with sensory experiences.

If you experience that Ishwara pranidhara,
maha bandha or pranayama is difficult to
practice, you can instead use different sensory
experiences such as sight, hearing, smell, taste
and touch to create a steady and calm mind.

Nada yoga (antar mouna)
Trataka
Kirtan
Mantra

36: 1

EXPERIENCE THE INNER LIGHT - OPTIONAL MEDITATION ON WHAT THE MIND IS DRAWN TO NATURALLY.

Viśokā vā jyotiṣmatī

Visoka: without sorrow, va: or, jyotismati: filled with light.

The state beyond grief when filled with light can control the mind.

The mind can also be calmed by experiencing the inner peace and light between the eyebrows, bhrumadhya or by nada, concentration on sound. This inner light is calm, still and peaceful and is experienced during deep meditation.

MEDITATION

Meditation aims to establish a contact with our inner self and increase our self-awareness. The goal is to realise ourselves. When a person achieves self-realisation, they have contact with their innermost self and identifies their existence – their life, based on their true self and not on the basis of their ego. During meditation, we try to establish an observed self, which means that we study our own thoughts objectively and neutrally. To thus gain a perspective on ourselves, our thoughts and feelings, and our existence.

It can be said that the purpose of meditation is to explore the different regions of the mind, learn how the mind works and train it to finally surpass the mind completely. In practical terms, it can be said that meditation is about emptying the mind of thoughts, by concentrating on the present through an activity or method.

ACTIVE MEDITATION
Active meditation means that we use breathing together with some form of movement in order to calm the thoughts and get into the present.

Examples of active meditation are yoga, qigong and tai chi. Active meditation can also be part of our everyday life in the form of walks, eating, etc, if you do it with presence. We learn how to put our feet up and breathe, how it feels in the body, and so on.

PASSIVE MEDITATION

Passive meditation – which most people may associate with meditation, means that we sit down in silence to practice some form of meditation technique. We train the mind through a specific method or technique to put ourselves in a meditative state.

PREPARATIONS

When sitting down for meditation, it is important to think about a few things. The first preparation is that you can sit undisturbed, in a place where you feel silence. Turn off all phones and make sure no one is disturbed. The morning or before bedtime are the best times for meditation. Also remember not to eat too close to the meditation, as the body is full of digestion and a lot of blood and energy is drawn in from the body to the stomach.

Then make sure you have something to sit on:
a meditation pillow, a regular pillow or a chair.
Take the time to find a comfortable sitting position. It is important that you sit comfortably
as you will sit still for a while. A popular sitting
position is siddhasana, where you sit on the
buttocks with the legs outstretched, insert one
foot towards the groin and the other foot you
place just in front of the shin or alternatively on
top of the shin. Make sure you are sitting in a
three-point position where both buttocks are in
contact with the ground and both knees.

You place your hands either on your knees with
the palm facing down and let your thumb and
forefinger meet in jnana mudra. Alternatively,
place the right back of the hand in the left palm
and let the thumbs meet in bhairavi mudra. It is
important that you feel your hands resting secu-
rely so that you can relax your shoulders.

Feel that you are sitting with a straight spine
where the weight from the upper body can fall
straight down through the pelvis. Tuck your
chin slightly to your chest so that your neck can
relax, and close your eyes. Shift a little weight
forward on the pelvis so that you do not collapse
with your back.

Then start by landing in yourself with your thoughts and with your presence, calm the mind and relax the body with, for example, kaya sthairyam. Then start your chosen meditation technique with, for example, ajapa japa. It is important not to have any expectations of the meditation and what we are believed to experience.

There are also various obstacles that you may encounter during meditation, such as thoughts and feelings. There can be obstacles such as anger, pride and selfishness, which can be trained away by practice yamas and niyamas. If any thoughts or feelings arise during the meditation, become aware of them, see them but then let them float on with the next exhalation and then return to focusing on the chosen meditation technique.

If you feel that it is difficult to calm down, it can be an advantage to have done something active before setting out for meditation, such as taking a walk or doing a yoga session.

It is important to have regularity in your meditation practice.

CLASSICAL TECHNIQUES FOR MEDITATION

The classic sitting positions for meditation (meditation asanas) are padmasana, siddhasana, siddha yoni asana and swastikasana. For beginners (and westerners who are often stiff and have narrower hips) you can also sit in sukhasana or ardha padmasana. If for various reasons you need to sit on a chair, you can also do so. The principle is that the sitting position should be comfortable and provide support for the body during meditation so you can relax. It's not about sitting nicely. It is important that the back is straight so that the prana can flow upwards in the body. You can also lie comfortably on your back, but then there is the risk of falling asleep.

Important mudras during a meditation include jnana / chin mudra, bhairavi mudra and khechari mudra.

JNANA MUDRA

Place your hands on your knees with your palms facing down and let your thumb and forefinger meet.

CHIN MUDRA

Place your hands on your knees with the palm facing up and let your thumb and forefinger meet.

BHAIRAVI MUDRA

Place the right back of the hand in the left palm and let your thumbs meet.

KHECHARI MUDRA

Roll up the tongue so that you place the back of the tongue up in the palate with a gentle pressure.

UJJAYI PRANAYAMA

Ujjayi pranayama also called the psychic / winning breath. Start by placing the back of the tongue up in the palate in the khechari mudra, narrow in the air passage and strive for a whispering / hissing ah sound. Breathe through your nose but feel that the breathing and the sound come far in from the throat. It sounds a bit like when you blow mist on a mirror with an open mouth. Children usually say that the sound is similar to Darth Vader's breathing in Star Wars.

Ujjayi pranayama is used in many different

meditation techniques (and also during the practice of asanas) as it has a calming effect on the nervous system and also lowers blood pressure. It also emits a sound as a focal point to draw attention to. Breathing in this way also means that you retain the heat.

BHRUMADHYA

Bhrumadhya is a point in the ajna chakra (third eye). The word itself, bhrumadhya, means eyebrow centre and this is also where this point is located.

CHIDAKASHA

Chidakasha can be explained as our inner mental television screen. It is visualised as a space in front of our closed eyes and this is where our psychic event appears – "what the mind carries". Chidakasha literally stands for "area of knowledge" and Akasha means space.

JAPA YOGA

Japa yoga is an effective technique for bringing the mind back to the present using the mantra. Japa means repetition of mantra. The mantra affects us both physically and mentally, both with the help of the meaning of the word and the vibrations it starts within one. Mantra meditation cleanses the subconscious mind and causes thought activity to decrease, as the mind does not receive any new stimulus. This makes it easier to get in touch with our inner self.

A constant repetition of the mantra makes the mind concentrated and relaxed and gives us inner peace. It is important not to force focus on the mantra but to let it come naturally from within. One can practice japa with different forms of mantras; they can be mantras that one pronounces aloud (baikhari), mantras to whisper (upanshu), mental mantras (mansaik), or written mantras (likhit). We often recite the mantra a certain number of times and to help us with the count you can have a mala, which is a string of beads. You can practice japa yoga both sitting in a meditation position or while performing other daily activities.

AJAPA JAPA

Ajapa japa is a complete sadhana (spiritual practice where one eventually achieves self-realisation) in itself. By regularly practicing ajapa japa for a long time, subconscious desires, fears will finally come to the surface which we will then view with a witness attitude. We thus get to the root of physical and mental problems and can change them.

Japa means repetition of mantra. Ajapa japa means constant awareness. Traditionally, the mantra So-Ham is used, but it is possible to use any mantra if, for example, you have received a mantra from your guru.

HARI OM TAT SAT

A guided meditation often ends with Hari Om Tat Sat in classical yoga.

Hari Om Tat Sat are actually two different mantras that have been brought together, Hari Om is one and Tat Sat is the other. Hari stands for the manifested universe and life, the energy – Shakti. Om stands for the absolute reality, the consciousness – Shiva. Reality consists of both the complete (incomprehensible) and the obvious, or the more concrete. This reality is presented in the mantra Hari Om Tat Sat. Satya means truth. Tat Sat means "it is the truth". Hari Om Tat Sat means both the concrete – what I can see – and the unknown or incomprehensible, which is also part of the same reality and not different.

YOGASCHITTA VRITTI NIRODHAH

(When the movements of the mind are still, yoga occurs)